Natural & Organic Beauty Recipes

A Complete Guide on Making Your Own Facial Masks, Toners, Lotions, Moisturizers, & Scrubs at Home with Simple & Easy Organic Skin Care Recipes

Evelyn R. Scott
Copyright© 2014 by Evelyn R. Scott

Natural & Organic Beauty Recipes

Copyright© 2014 Evelyn R. Scott

All Rights Reserved.

Warning: The unauthorized reproduction or distribution of this copyrighted work is illegal. No part of this book may be scanned, uploaded or distributed via internet or other means, electronic or print without the author's permission. Criminal copyright infringement without monetary gain is investigated by the FBI and is punishable by up to 5 years in federal prison and a fine of $250,000. (http://www.fbi.gov/ipr/). Please purchase only authorized electronic or print editions and do not participate in or encourage the electronic piracy of copyrighted material.

Publisher: Enlightened Publishing

ISBN-13: 978-1499234305

ISBN-10: 1499234309

Disclaimer

The Publisher has strived to be as accurate and complete as possible in the creation of this book. While all attempts have been made to verify information provided in this publication, the Publisher assumes no responsibility for errors, omissions, or contrary interpretation of the subject matter herein. Any perceived slights of specific persons, peoples, or organizations are unintentional.

This book is not intended for use as a source of legal, business, accounting or financial advice. All readers are advised to seek services of competent professionals in the legal, business, accounting, and finance fields.

The information in this book is not intended or implied to be a substitute for professional medical advice, diagnosis or treatment. All content contained in this book is for general information purposes only. Always consult your healthcare provider before carrying on any health program.

Table of Contents

Introduction 3

Chapter 1: The Ugly Truth behind Commercial Skin Care Products 7

    Ingredients to Avoid 8
    Other Questionable Ingredients 15
    What's Really Organic? 18

Chapter 2: All about Your Skin 21

    Oily Skin 22
    Dry Skin 23
    Combination Skin 24
    Sensitive Skin 25
    Aging Skin 26
    Skin-Care Tips 28

Chapter 3: Making Your Own Organic Skin Care Treatments 33

    Natural Ingredients 35
    Tips for Making Your Own Products 42

Chapter 4: Applying Skin Care Treatments.. 45

    Cleanser 46

    Toner 47

    Moisturizer 47

    Scrub 49

    Mask 50

    Eye Treatments 51

Chapter 5: Moisturizer Recipes 53

Chapter 6: Facial Mask Recipes 67

Chapter 7: Facial Toner Recipes 81

Chapter 8: Facial Scrub Recipes 95

Chapter 9: Eye Treatment Recipes 109

Introduction

Women around the world spend billions of dollars every year on beauty products. They buy soaps to clean their skin, tonics to tighten their pores, lotions to add moisture and scrubs and masks to perform miracles like erasing wrinkles and eliminating puffy eyes.

Because they know there are billions to be made, beauty product manufacturers create new formulas all the time, each one promising to achieve better results than the last. The problem is, many of the products sold at drug stores or at cosmetic counters contain chemically derived ingredients that have actually been found to irritate the skin, do the opposite of what they say, and even cause cancer.

In addition, they are horribly expensive. You can purchase a jar of nighttime face cream that is said to include bits of gold and costs more than $200. Does it work? There is no way to know until you try it.

But instead of subject yourself to dangerous ingredients or emptying your wallet, you can actually make many beauty products with natural ingredients that you probably already have in your kitchen. These can cost just a few cents to make and are just as, if not more, effective than creams that costs hundreds of dollars.

In this guide, you will learn some of the common ingredients that the beauty industry subjects you to, why they are dangerous, and what to look for on labels if you choose to buy your beauty products over-the-counter.

You will also learn how to determine what kind of skin you have—dry, oily, combination or sensitive—and which natural ingredients will help to counteract the effects of your natural skin type.

Also included are the basics of natural skin-care ingredients and what type of daily and weekly beauty regime you should follow to achieve your most beautiful, youthful, and glowing complexion. You will learn which natural ingredients—from bananas to oatmeal to olive oil—will help you achieve better skin tone, fewer wrinkles, and better hydrated skin. There are even plenty of tips for day-to-day lifestyle changes that can have a direct effect on the appearance of your skin (such as beauty sleep and stress reduction).

You will also find 50 recipes and step-by-step-instructions for inexpensive, natural skincare formulas that take only minutes to mix up, will save you a lot of money over time, and keep you safe from the irritating, cancer-causing ingredients found in everyday skincare products on the market.

You can naturally and easily improve your skin without spending a fortune. Read on to learn more.

Chapter 1: The Ugly Truth behind Commercial Skin Care Products

The quest for more beautiful skin has many of us heading to the local drug store or cosmetics counter for answers. Which formula will cleanse my face the best? Do I need an exfoliating product? How can I get my wrinkles to look less pronounced? Sound familiar? We are so concerned about the end result that we don't stop to think, "What is actually in this $50 jar of face cream?"

While the U.S. Food and Drug Administration (FDA) requires skin-care product makers to list all of the ingredients on the product's label, it might be impossible to make sense of them. What in the world is ethylhexylglycerin or polyglycryl-2 dipolyhydroxystearate? It is almost as if these ingredient names are made to be as confusing as possible so you will just purchase the product on the promise that you will achieve more glowing skin or fewer visible wrinkles in a month.

Companies include these ingredients to do a number of things: make them smell better, make them last longer, and make them less expensive and easier to manufacture. While these may be beneficial to the companies that are making them, many of the ingredients have been shown to irritate the skin, damage the eyes, wreak havoc with internal hormones, and possibly even lead to cancer.

While the products are not controlled by the FDA, some of the formulas still include these dangerous ingredients. As the general public becomes more aware of the harmful effects of these ingredients, some of the biggest beauty brands are becoming involved in a movement towards more natural and organic formulas.

Ingredients to Avoid

Which are some of the ingredients you should know about? Here are 14 that are considered to be dangerous and should be avoided:

- **Synthetic polymers**. You can find this gelling agent in all sorts of products like shampoo, skin creams, and makeup. They are also used to create plastics and glue. These are widely used and have many manufacturing applications, but are considered toxic if absorbed into the skin. They'll be listed as sodium polyacrylate or carbomer in the ingredients.

- **Sulfates**. If you like to work up a lather with your shampoo or facial cleanser, chances are that you are using products that include lots of sulfates. These are considered harsh cleansing agents and thickeners that do indeed help to remove dirt, but will also sting the eyes. People with a low tolerance for sulfates may experience headaches, hives, or worse. Sulfates have been linked to premature baldness, cataract formation, certain forms of cancer, and vision problems for children. Look for ingredient names like sodium lauryl or sodium laureth.

- **Synthetic fragrances**. Yes, we all like to smell nice, but a large portion of the population is sensitive to artificial scents. About 5 percent cannot tolerate them at all and another 30 percent are sensitive to these fragrances. Headaches are fairly common, but people with asthma may experience an asthma attack and some synthetic fragrances are suspected of damaging organs like the kidneys and liver. Toluene and phthalates are some of the chemicals used to make synthetic fragrances, and they can disrupt hormones or cause developmental problems. A better option is to use those that are created from natural essential oils.

- **Parabens**. You may notice more and more products labels that alert you to the fact that they are "paraben-free." That is because these antimicrobial chemicals, which are used as product preservatives, actually mimic the hormone estrogen and are considered to be influential in the increase of breast cancer cases. Watch out for ingredients that end with "paraben," like ethylparaben or butylparaben.

- **Synthetic colors.** Don't be fooled by the pretty mint or baby pink of your favorite beauty product. Ingredients like FD&C or D&C are synthetic colors, usually listed as a color followed by a number, like FD&C blue 1, are often derived from coal tar that may include cancer-causing agents. Some of these, like Red #3, have actually been banned by the FDA because of its link to cancer, but many others still remain on the market.

- **Triethanolamine (TEA).** This ingredient is often used to balance the pH in skin moisturizers, mascara, and shampoos at all different price points, from simple drug store formulas to department store luxury products. It can be irritating to the eyes or skin and may even spark allergic reactions. Studies have found evidence of cancer in animals exposed to TEA. Similar ingredients include diethanolamines (DEA) and coconut oil amide of monoethanolamine (MEA).

- **Stearalkonium chloride.** This chemical was originally developed as a fabric softener to fight static cling, but manufacturers found that it was a cheap alternative for hair conditioners as well. At higher concentrations, this ingredient shows adverse effects around the eyes and mouth but since the labels don't tell you at what percentage the concentration is, how could you know?

- **Urea**. As you may guess from its name, this ingredient was once formulated from horse urine and included in beauty products because of its skin-softening benefits. It is not synthetically created and is often used as a preservative. It is listed as diazolidinyl urea or imidazolidinyl urea, although you may see them on labels as Germall II or Germall 115. The last two are forms of urea combined with other preservatives in order to increase effectiveness.

- **Petrolatum**. This is one ingredient that the beauty industry has fooled you into thinking is actually beneficial for moisturizing the skin. In truth, it is derived from petroleum and just sits on the surface never actually penetrating the skin. While petrolatum itself is not considered particularly harmful, it is easily contaminated with certain hydrocarbons during the manufacturing process that are believed to cause cancer and reproductive toxicity. So why do the manufacturers use it? They use it because the public believes that it moisturizes and protects the skin (it doesn't), and because it is cheap.

- **Propylene glycol**. You can find this mineral oil in all sorts of beauty products, like skin cream, bubble bath, after shave, and makeup, but you can also find it in paint, wallpaper stripper, antifreeze, and tire sealant. While it may work to seal in moisture, it is also very irritating to the skin and may cause damage to the liver or kidneys. It is easily absorbed into the skin and can cause damage on a cellular level.

- **PVP/VA Copolymer**. If you have ever used a hair styling product, chances are that it contained this glue-like ingredient. The chemical is derived from petroleum, and is considered to be harmful to the lungs if inhaled. So either try to hold your breath while using your hairspray and hope it all dissipates...or avoid it altogether.

- **1,4-dioxane**. This ingredient is practically omnipresent throughout the world of skin-care supplies since it is processed with petroleum-based ethylene oxide. But its effects are widespread, from irritating the eyes to acting as a depressant on the central nervous system. It can cause headaches and dizziness and, if inhaled, can harm the liver and kidneys, and even lead to blood disorders. It is often listed on ingredient labels in words that end in "-eth), like myreth or laureth.

- **Alcohol**. Some forms of alcohol used in beauty products (which is different from the type of alcohol that you drink), can be extremely irritating to the skin. Alcohol may be included in skin-care products like toners or acne pads, and seem to give a tightening or tingling effect that feels like it is "doing something." However, this is not beneficial for those with sensitive skin as moisture will be wicked out and the user will be left with dry skin. As dry skin typically leads to prematurely aged skin, these effects are better to avoid. The types of alcohol in these products that are of particular concern include ethanol, methanol, SD alcohol, alcohol denat, or isopropyl alcohol, which can lead to brown spots on the skin.

- **Benzalkonium chloride**. This is an antiseptic that has been very closely monitored in cosmetics in other countries, yet is still found in many sprays and topical products. It is known to irritate the skin, eyes, and even the lungs if inhaled. While it is effective in eliminating micro-organisms, the effects of benzalkonium chloride are unknown for pregnant women and their unborn babies.

Other Questionable Ingredients

While other ingredients may not be as toxic as the mostly synthetic chemicals listed above, some may simply be misleading. Here's a sampling:

- **Collagen**. This is a protein substance found naturally within the structure of the skin. It is what helps to give the skin its volume, which makes for a more youthful complexion and fewer wrinkles. However, as people age, collagen production diminishes. Upon this discovery, the beauty industry decided to start adding collagen to topical products. The problem is, topical collagen is too large to actually penetrate the skin and be absorbed. Therefore, expensive creams that promise to add collagen to the skin do nothing but sit on top of the skin and trap bacteria and dead skin cells. A better approach is to use ingredients that actually promote collagen production at a cellular level or consume foods that boost collagen production (more on that later).

- **Elastin**. This is another protein naturally found in skin tissue that diminishes as we age. It is included in some beauty products with promises that it will help to firm the skin. However, like collagen, it cannot be absorbed through the outer layer of skin; therefore it has no effect when applied topically.

- **Glycerin**. You will find this ingredient, or some form of it, on nearly every topical beauty product that is sold. It is created by mixing water and fat to draw the glycerin out of the fat. While it is said to act as a moisturizer, it actually draws moisture out of the skin. The real purpose of adding glycerin to a cream or lotion is to make the products easier to smooth across your skin.

- **Mineral oil**. This is a confusing one, because "mineral" sounds organic. However, it is typically created from crude oil. Mineral oil is a major cause of allergic reactions and acne breakouts, and is another substance that simply does not absorb well into the outer surface of the skin. Further, it interferes with the natural oils found within your skin and can create surface-level dryness.

What's Really Organic?

Since the general public has become increasingly aware of the dangerous chemicals and misleading ingredients included in skincare formulas, "organic" and "natural" options have populated the market. While that may seem a promising advancement to ensure people are not exposed to cancer-causing ingredients, the truth is that these products are not regulated by any government agency.

Even though a product may say "organic" or "natural" on the label, that might be because it includes one or two untainted ingredients along with whatever else the manufacture has decided to use. The most common problem with truly organic products is that they have shorter shelf-lives than those that are chemically engineered. To solve this, the manufacturer adds a preservative to make your product last longer.

The U.S. Department of Agriculture has created a voluntary certification program so that companies can label their ingredients to better help consumers choose the products that are right for them. The certifications include:

- **"100% Organic."** These must include only organic ingredients that have not been chemically altered, with the exception of water and salt.

- **"Organic."** These must include 95 percent organic ingredients and the other 5 percent must be those that are on the USDA approved list.

- **"Made with organic ingredients."** These must include at least three organic ingredients listed on the label and make up to no less than 70 percent of the products ingredients.

Any products that fall below those numbers are not certified to be called "organic," but again, there is no agency that is regulating these products and their ingredients, so you still may be fooled into buying fake "organic" products. Look for the green and white seal that says "USDA Organic" to be sure.

Chapter 2: All about Your Skin

The skin on your face is different than the rest of your body's skin. It is typically more sensitive and reacts more strongly to hormonal changes. Plus, as we age, we become hyper-focused on what is happening to the structure of our skin. Namely: fine lines, volume loss, sagging and wrinkling.

The first step in determining what type of skin-care products you need to maintain a healthy-looking complexion is to figure out what type of skin you have and how it reacts under challenging circumstances. The main types are oily, dry, combination, sensitive, and aging skin. Here is how to tell what you are dealing with:

Oily Skin

You may think that people with oily skin are the only ones who suffer from acne, but it may be some consolation to know that acne can affect all skin types. It is true, however, that those with oily skin may be more susceptible to acne thanks to an over-production of sebum.

Sebum is the oil that is naturally excreted from the sebaceous glands in the skin. If it comes into contact with dead skin cells that haven't been cleared from the skin along with bacteria, a pimple may form. People with oily skin have an excess of sebum, which will need to be properly controlled.

Many oily-skin sufferers think they need to clean their skin more often, and with harsher astringents, than those with less-oily skin types. Excessive cleansing can not only strip your skin of the necessary levels of sebum, but may also lead to dehydrated skin, which is different from dry skin.

Skin can become dehydrated in all skin types and simply means that the skin is in need of moisture. Often people with oily skin mistakenly think they shouldn't use a moisturizer. Nothing could be further from the truth. Dehydrated skin likes to hold on to dead skin cells and this promotes the growth of blemishes. Choosing an appropriate moisturizer is key for oily-skin. Aloe vera is an ideal natural ingredient for helping oily skin types to achieve better balance.

Dry Skin

If the surface of your skin seems ashy or if it feels particularly tight after cleansing, you may have dry skin. Dry skin is lacking in natural hydration and, as oily skin is prone to acne, is prone to red patches and prematurely developed fine lines and wrinkles.

Dry skin can become irritated easily and is particularly sensitive during the winter months and to climates that are low in humidity. This is when the skin may become more red and itchy.

The temptation may be to moisturize excessively with lotions and creams, but, of course, some of these will not even penetrate your skin, and while you may be temporarily relieved of symptoms, these products sit on the surface and suffocate your skin. Plus, the dead skin cells on the surface can't be eliminated and you may find yourself suffering from breakouts.

Natural moisturizers that include oatmeal, shea butter or coconut oil can help to add needed soothing while not clogging your pores. You can also try running a humidifier in your home to help to add moisture to the air…and your skin.

Combination Skin

This can be the most difficult to control because different areas of the face have different levels of oil and dryness. Those people with combination skin often see more oily and shiny skin along their foreheads and down their nose and chin, known as the T-zone. The sebaceous glands are simply more active here.

Dry skin is often found along the cheeks, jowls, and eye areas. Unfortunately, people with combination skin are prone to all of the various skin woes like acne, redness, and premature aging in the form of fine lines and wrinkles.

A smart approach to this two-toned skin type is to use a gel moisturizer that will nourish your dry skin and not clog the pores of your oily skin, as well as a natural toner along the T-zone. When problems arise, such as wrinkles or acne, you may want to spot treat only those areas with products geared to help those particular problems—for instance, use a super-hydrating cream around dry eyes and a bacteria-reducing formula for intermittent breakouts.

Sensitive Skin

If you have sensitive skin you most likely already know because it is easily irritated if you use a new product or enter extreme conditions, like very cold or very warm weather, or areas where there is a lot of environmental pollution. You may be born with dry or oily skin, and eventually wind up with very sensitive skin that is prone to redness, discomfort, itchiness, broken blood vessels in the face, excessive blushing, or occasional dryness.

People with chronically sensitive skin may suffer from rosacea or eczema, which makes the skin red and itchy, while others may only have occasional sensitivity caused by products or certain ingredients.

Opting for more natural products will need to be done gradually (as will making any other changes to your skin care) because drastic changes may cause harsh skin reactions. Introduce new products or ingredients slowly. Those with sensitive skin will most certainly want to avoid any chemical ingredients like synthetic fragrances or colors, as well as alcohol, as it is particularly drying.

Aging Skin

No matter what type of skin you have, it will eventually age, bringing a host of additional skin-care concerns. With age, a few key things start to happen within the structure of the skin: Collagen production slows. This protein naturally found in the skin helps its volume, and with less of it the face starts losing its fullness. This is particularly troublesome because your facial expressions will eventually start to create folds and wrinkles that become permanent as the amount of collagen decreases.

Aging skin will also start to lose its youthful glow as cellular regeneration starts to slow. This will lead to more dead skin cells on the surface of your skin, which can give you an ashy or gray skin tone that lacks the vibrancy your skin once held. Making good, healthy food choices can help to improve your skin at a cellular level (and it can help with collagen production, too).

Because dead skin cells are particularly present in aging skin, regular exfoliation is necessary to reveal the fresh skin below. Using a scrub made of natural ingredients is an ideal way to slough away dulling dead skin, and will also ensure that you are not exposing your delicate skin to harsh chemicals found in many aggressive exfoliation products found on the market.

Another thing to keep in mind is that as you lose weight, it will show in your face. While a loss of fat in your body may be the goal, losing fat in your face can actually make you appear older. Aim for a healthy, not too low, body weight and keep your skin healthy and glowing to avoid a prematurely aged-looking face.

Skin-Care Tips

Once you have conquered the problems associated with your particular skin type there are some overall tips for healthy-looking skin that everyone can follow. Here's how to take care of your skin on a regular basis:

- **Cleanse**. Wash your face with a gentle cleanser morning and night. If you have dry or combination skin, you may want to only clean your face at night to remove the day's makeup.

- **Moisturize**. Find a hydrating formula that includes ingredients geared for your skin type and use it twice a day. Your skin needs moisture to create the soft, dewy look that we all strive for.

- **Exfoliate**. Use a gentle scrub twice a week to remove any dead skin cells that might be lingering and clogging your pores or making your skin look dull. Once you begin exfoliating regularly, you will notice that your other products work better, you will not need to use them as frequently, and your makeup looks better.

- **Use a mask**. If you need some extra pampering, use a mask once a week or every other week. Unlike a scrub that works to remove dead skin cells, a mask will add in essential nutrients that your facial skin will soak up.

- **Be gentle**. Stop using any product that stings or feels harsh. Don't tug on your skin and when you cleanse and exfoliate, use the tips of your fingers and gently massage with slow, circular motions

- **Wear sunscreen**. Nothing will age your skin faster than exposing it to the sun without proper protection. If you go without sunscreen, you can be sure that you will have wrinkles sooner, as well as unsightly dark spots on your face, hands, and chest. Plus you are putting yourself at risk for skin cancer. Look for sunscreens that are chemical-free, especially when using it on your face. Many brands of makeup also include sunscreen in their formulas. You can further protect your skin by wearing a wide-brim hat.

- **Eat right**. Certain foods are full of skin-boosting antioxidants that help at a cellular level and even help to boost collagen production. Some of the best options are red and orange fruits and vegetables (berries, carrots, sweet potatoes, tomatoes, peppers, beets), veggies that contain large amounts of water (cucumbers, celery), dark green veggies (kale, spinach, collard greens), omega-3-rich foods (fatty fish, walnuts, olive oil), and tea (white, green).

- **Eliminate damaging foods**. Prepackaged, processed foods (think: bagged potato chips, cookies, pastas and others) as well as foods that include a lot of sugar have been shown to increase inflammation. This causes your body to take longer to heal and can make skin conditions like acne and rosacea even worse and more difficult to treat. Clean the bad carbohydrates and sugary foods out of your diet and your skin will soon be looking and feeling better.

- **Reduce stress**. This will also increase inflammation within your body and cause hormones to go out of whack, which can lead to blemishes. Exercising regularly and scheduling massages once a month can do wonders to both combat stress and the effects it has on your skin. To get an extra-rosy boost, take a brisk walk every morning and you will start to see some healthy color in your cheeks.

- **Get sleep**. They don't call it beauty sleep for nothing. Getting adequate rest every night (six to eight hours) will help to revitalize your skin, improve its elasticity, and repair any damages. Plus, sleep is a great way to avoid under-eye puffiness.

- **Quit smoking**. Smoking wicks moisture out of the skin and causes a depletion of vitamin C which is critical for collagen and elastin production. Plus, people who smoke are more likely to develop tiny, vertical lines above their top lip which are very difficult to reverse.

- **Change your sheets often**. Bacteria can build up on your pillow case and eventually make its way onto your skin, where it can clog pores and cause breakouts.

- **Drink water regularly**. If there is just one thing you do to help your skin, it is to drink more water. Hydrating your skin from the inside out will make a dramatic difference in the appearance and overall health of your skin. Aim for at least eight glasses per day and always drink a glass of water after consuming dehydrating beverages like coffee, tea or alcohol.

Chapter 3: Making Your Own Organic Skin Care Treatments

There are many valid reasons to want to make your own skin-care products, but most people opt for creating their own formulas to either save money or to avoid the harsh, irritating, cancer-causing chemicals that many beauty industry manufacturers use in their products.

You can pay up to $200 for a jar of moisturizer from an elitist company that is simply banking on their profits. Their product, however, may not be providing you with the type of skin-care that your unique complexion needs. For mere pennies, you can make a naturally fragrant, soothing moisturizer that you know will help to hydrate your skin because you are in charge of which ingredients you are using.

Reading the label of any given beauty product is like trying to decipher a foreign language and it is unlikely that you even know what the ingredients mean. A good rule of thumb, by the way, is: **If you wouldn't eat it, don't put it on your skin.** Your skin is your body's largest organ and it serves the very important task of protecting your body from many traumas and assaults. Why would you want to slather on a chemical that you cannot even pronounce onto this vital protective organ?

Many of the chemically derived formulas that the beauty industry makes are formulated from what started out as natural ingredients. Why not use the natural ingredient to begin with and get results that are just as effective, if not more so, than expensive beauty products?

Making your own skin-care products is a great way to avoid such chemicals, because it is unlikely that you will be able to get your hands on any stearalkonium chloride or triethanolamine. It is easier to find more scrumptious ingredients like honey, bananas, yogurt, cucumbers, coffee, herbs, ginger, eggs, milk, and more.

Natural Ingredients

Just like these wholesome foods and ingredients can help your body and skin from the inside out, they also have healing and protective properties when used topically on your skin. Here's how they can help:

- **Oatmeal**. No longer just for breakfast, this morning-meal staple is actually very versatile when used as a skin-care ingredient. It can soothe a sunburn, relieve dryness, help the skin to retain moisture, reduce odor, and remove dirt. It can also be used in cleansers, scrubs or masks.

- **Honey**. This is another all-purpose natural ingredient that will hydrate and soothe your skin. It can also ease inflammation, such as acne, on contact, and reduce bacteria. Because of its smooth texture and sweet scent, you will find it in many homemade beauty product recipes.

- **Bananas**. Sufferers of dry skin will find that mashed up bananas go a long way to soothe their skin as well as add lots of moisture while the antioxidants help to naturally promote collagen production. They are particularly helpful in easing cracked dry skin on the feet. Plus, they are inexpensive and generally available all year round.

- **Herbs**. Many cultures have used various herbs for their medicinal properties and for their ability to enhance beauty. Turmeric is used to promote glowing skin in face masks. Rosemary is believed to revitalize at a cellular level. Chamomile is often added to eye creams for its anti-inflammatory properties. Evening primrose is often used to heal various skin conditions. Because they can be chopped or ground, they are easy to mix into recipes.

- **Ginger**. This super-fragrant antioxidant and anti-inflammatory can help to soothe dry skin, work as an effective exfoliator in scrubs, and can even help to reduce white spots on the skin when rubbed on daily.

- **Sugar**. Although consuming sugar is known to wreak havoc on skin because it worsens inflammation, it is actually a helpful ingredient to use topically. Because it contains glycolic acid, it works as a good skin moisturizer and can protect the skin from toxins. Its texture is also perfect for helping to slough away dead skin cells when used in a scrub. White or brown sugar will work, depending on your preference.

- **Yogurt**. This creamy ingredient is great to use as a base as it will help to smooth on other ingredients. It will also help make your pores appear smaller and is an excellent natural exfoliant because it includes lactic acid.

- **Olive oil**. The use of olive oil as a beauty product goes back to Cleopatra's days. It is believed to be super hydrating for most skin types, but it is best to use in the evenings when you are not wearing makeup. Men with sensitive skin may also want to apply olive oil before shaving to avoid the harsh chemicals in shaving creams. It is also a great mixing agent for scrubs and, in a pinch, can help you remove stubborn makeup.

- **Cucumbers**. You have probably seen women receiving spa treatments with slices of cucumbers on their eyes. That is because they are believed to reduce under-eye puffiness. Cucumber is used in facial masks to soothe irritated skin, and also works well as a toner because it is a natural astringent.

- **Coffee**. This may be your morning boost, but coffee is also known for its many beauty benefits. Caffeine is believed to help reduce cellulite as well as constrict the blood vessels that cause rosacea and dark under-eye circles. The texture of ground coffee is also ideal for creating scrubs when mixed with an oil, like olive oil.

- **Eggs**. This breakfast staple is not only versatile in the kitchen, but can also be adaptably used beauty-wise. It can help achieve better shine for dry hair and egg whites can help to tighten the skin. When used as a facial mask, it can reduce blemishes and create a more healthful glow.

- **Milk**. This nourishing beauty ingredient is known to hydrate the skin and help with cellular renewal. It may also help to ease redness and create a glowing complexion. Because it contains lactic acid, milk may also be included in natural exfoliating scrubs that cleanse and nourish the skin from the outside, in.

- **Rose water**. This is a lovely ingredient to add to your beauty routine because of its natural floral scent. It is also a great astringent, making it useful in toners and cleansers. Keep some in a spritzer to relieve sunburns, or even eliminate body odors. You can buy 100% rose water in health food stores or make your own by simmering rose petals in water.

- **Peaches**. There is a reason people refer to a healthy complexion as "peachy." The fruit is not only the color of a beautiful skin tone, but peach juice may also help to unclog pores, lighten age spots, and even reduce wrinkles when included in moisturizers or masks. You can even simply rub the peach flesh onto your skin, wait a few minutes, and then rinse with warm water for a dewy complexion.

- **Lemon**. You may have used lemon juice as a teen to lighten your hair in the sun. Now, you might consider using lemon to remove age spots on your skin or to whiten yellowed fingernails, which is effective. This is due to the fruit's high levels of vitamin C, which is used in many over-the-counter age-spot removers. Lemons can be irritating, so use conservatively until you see how your skin reacts to it.

- **Pumpkin**. This is a wonderfully fragrant squash that is packed with lots of skin-saving vitamins, including vitamin C, E, A, and beta carotene. You get all of these antioxidants right on your face when you mix pumpkin into a mask or scrub. It will help to refresh your skin and clear out your pores.

- **Aloe vera**. Many skin-care product manufacturers use aloe vera in their formulas because of its ability to reduce under-eye puffiness, soothe irritations, moisturize chapped lips, and reduce blemishes. If you have access to a plant, you will see that its juices are readily available if you cut the leaf.

- **Almonds**. Almonds can be used in a variety of forms to enhance your at-home beauty routine. You can grind almonds in a coffee grinder and then use them in a scrub to help naturally exfoliate your skin. You may also want to try almond oil, which naturally contains linoleic acid, known to moisturize the skin. Eating almonds is also believed to benefit the skin, thanks to their antioxidants and healthy fats.

- **Sea salt**. This ingredient is an unrefined salt that is full of vitamins and minerals that are essential for good health. It is super soothing when used topically and is the perfect consistency to use as a scrub when mixed with honey, almond oil, or olive oil. It can also be a revitalizing addition to your bath.

Tips for Making Your Own Products

Fresh, organic ingredients spoil more quickly than store-bought products, so you may want to make your at-home beauty products in small batches. If you make enough for more than one use, you should keep it in your refrigerator for no more than a week, then throw it out. You can always give them to a friend or invite someone over for an at-home spa day if you wind up with extras.

Recipes that last longer can be stored in dark containers and kept out of the sunlight. Also, when using your natural products, be sure to do so with clean, dry fingers, as water can contaminate your recipes.

You may want to experiment with different formulations to create scents that you like…and avoid ones that you don't.

Keep in mind that you will need to mix dry ingredients with something liquid in order to be able to apply it to your skin. Many homemade beauty products contain oils like olive or almond, or honey and yogurt especially for this purpose. The benefit is that all of those ingredients contain skin-boosting benefits too.

Because the ingredients are natural, their texture may vary for time to time. Experiment and don't be afraid to mix and match ingredients to suit your personal preferences and needs.

Chapter 4: Applying Skin Care Treatments

Now that you have explored the different types of homemade beauty product ingredients, you will want to decide which ones that you want to make. For healthy skin, you will want to follow a regime of daily cleaning, toning, and moisturizing, as well as occasional masks and scrubs to keep your pores clear and your skin well nourished.

Because you are using homemade products, know that some of the ingredients, like bananas or avocados, are going to be messier than your traditional creams and lotions. Be sure to set aside enough time to mix, apply and clean up your ingredients. It may seem like extra work, but you will be saving a lot of money and lessening the risk of exposing yourself to toxic chemicals. It is worth the extra effort.

In addition to making the products with natural ingredients, you will need a few other items, such as cotton balls or pads, a wash cloth, and a dry towel. You may also want to use Q-tips when applying small amounts of your eye treatments.

Cleanser

Because water alone won't properly wash your face, you need a cleanser to remove the majority of makeup, dirt, and grime we are subjected to every day. The best way to cleanse your face is to use warm water, which will help soften the face and allow for some gentle exfoliation when you wash your face.

When applying the cleanser, use your fingertips to gently massage the cleanser into your face with circular movements for about 30 seconds, being careful not to tug on the skin. Rinse the product with warm water and then use a washcloth to ensure that you have removed all of the product. Finish by patting your face dry with a towel, but not rubbing, which can eventually harm the skin.

Toner

To further clear out your pores and remove stubborn dirt and makeup that may have settled into your skin, a natural astringent—a toner—can help. Some people believe that a toner will shrink your pores, but that is not actually possible. You can reduce the appearance of your pores by ensuring that they are clear of dead skin cells and debris, but they will always be the same size you were born with.

People who have excessively oily skin can benefit the most from toners because they'll help to clear out debris and impurities that can eventually lead to pimples. Those with dry skin may be able to skip using a toner. To use a toner, first wash your face and then apply the toner gently with a cotton ball or pad. People with combination skin should focus on the T-zone and avoid the eye areas and cheeks.

Moisturizer

There is a lot of confusion about how to apply moisturizers. How much do you need, and how often should you do it? Moisturizers are important because they help our skin to retain moisture, which will improve its appearance and stave off the effects of dehydrated or dry skin, such as the formation of wrinkles. They also act as a protective barrier for the skin.

The ideal time to apply a moisturizer is immediately after cleansing, and using a toner. The skin should be slightly damp so that the moisturizer can do its work: trap the moisture in the skin. It is best to avoid the eye area, because this moisturizing action can make the skin around the eyes appear puffy.

Many moisturizers contain sun protection, which is good to use in the morning, but avoid an SPF when applying moisturizer at night. Don't forget to use your moisturizer on your neck, since the skin there is sensitive to the effects of aging. And if you have some extra, go ahead and massage it into your hands, which can always benefit from some extra hydration. Let your moisturizer dry completely before you move on to applying makeup.

Scrub

A facial scrub is important because even though you may be cleansing and using a toner, they may not remove all of the dead skin cells that can settle into your pores and lead to dull or blemished skin. Since you are mixing your own, you may want to experiment with certain scrubbing ingredients like sugar, salt, ground almonds, oatmeal, or others to decide which one feels the best on your face.

You may be tempted to use a scrub every day, but if you do so you may actually strip away the healthy oils that your skin makes naturally. These oils are essential in producing a healthy glow and helping your skin to retain moisture. If you have dry or combination skin, you should use an exfoliating scrub no more than once a week. Oilier skin types may want to use the scrub twice a week—but no more than that.

A good time to use a scrub is after you have been in the shower for a few minutes, so that the warm water has softened your skin. To use your scrub, wet your skin with warm water, then scoop up some of the scrub and gently massage it into your face, making small circular motions with the tips of your fingers.

If you have oily skin, you can scrub a bit more aggressively in your T-zone, but overall you will want to be gentle. Don't forget your neck and cleavage area too. Rinse the scrub off and pat your face dry with a towel.

Mask

A facial mask can serve several purposes. It can add nutrients and moisture to your skin, help to detoxify your skin, and soothe irritated skin. You will need to set aside up to 30 minutes to fully complete the process, so be sure to do it when you have some time to relax. It may seem like a once-in-a-while indulgence, but you can actually apply a facial mask a few times a week.

Apply the mask with your fingertips on a clean, dry face, avoiding the delicate skin around your eyes and lips. While you are waiting for the recommended time, try to relax by lying down and listening to some soothing music. Wash it off with a warm washcloth and pat your face dry with a towel.

If you have combination skin, consider applying the mask only to your T-zone. Those with sensitive skin may want to test the mask on a small area of skin to see if any irritation develops. Although you are using natural products, some fruit or vegetable enzymes can be irritating to sensitive skin.

Eye Treatments

The skin around your eyes needs moisture just like the rest of your skin, but because it is more delicate, you will want to give it special attention. When using an eye treatment, apply only a tiny bit with the tips of your ring fingers. Dab it gently under your eyes and wherever you can see fine lines forming, such as crow's-feet.

Because the skin is so easily damaged, you will want to apply the eye treatment with a patting motion rather than a rubbing motion, which can worsen under-eye puffiness and dark circles. Allow to absorb and dry before applying makeup.

Chapter 5: Moisturizer Recipes

Moisturizers serve one purpose: to add moisture to your skin. Unfortunately, you cannot simply add water, because it will eventually dry. Naturally made moisturizers can work as well, or even better, than store-bought ones and cost far less, as moisturizers are some of the most expensive products out there. In fact, by using these homemade versions, you may only need to spend about $20 for an entire year's supply.

If you have used commercial moisturizers, you are probably used to applying them and leaving them on. Some of the homemade recipes will be a bit richer, so you will want to wash them off. Don't worry; the ingredients will have done their job of locking in the moisture on your skin.

With some of these recipes, you can leave on the moisturizer for several hours to reap the benefits of the formulas. Try using those recipes on the weekends or at a time when you don't have to rush off somewhere, so that you can allow them to seep in for some time before rinsing them off.

To lock in the moisture, you will be using natural oils. Some work better for certain skin types than others. For instance, rich oils like olive oil or sesame oil may be best for dry skin types, but you will want to go for lighter oils, such as grapeseed or avocado, for combination or oily skin. If you find one you particularly like, and you need a moisturizer in a pinch, simply using a small amount of the oil on its own, smoothed over your face, will give you instant moisturizing protection.

Many of the ingredients found in these recipes you probably already have in your kitchen, but you may need to add some moisturizer-making staples such as beeswax and various oils. When making moisturizers you will often use natural oils, as well as an emulsifying wax, such as beeswax, which has been found to be compatible with human skin. These waxes will work to boost your skin's natural hydrating actions.

To make a moisturizer, you typically need an oil and an emulsifier that acts as a bonding ingredient to keep oil and other ingredients, like water, from separating. If you add solid oils (butters like cocoa or shea), your recipe will be thicker. If it is too thick, add some water. (Distilled water is best.)

You can add some natural fragrance by using a few drops of essential oil. These are available at your local health food store, and come in a wide variety of scents to choose from. Start with just a drop or two to determine how they interact with your other ingredients. Some of the best essential oils for facial recipes are chamomile for de-puffing, and rose for its moisturizing effects. Citrus oils or "fragrance" essential oils can cause irritation on sensitive skin.

Before applying the moisturizer, be sure that your face has been cleaned and that you have used a toner if you have oily skin. It is best to apply a moisturizer to slightly damp skin.

Cocoa butter moisturizer

Ingredients:

- 2 tablespoons beeswax, grated
- 1/2 cup cocoa butter
- 2 teaspoons water
- 1 tablespoon extra virgin olive oil
- 2 tablespoons coconut oil
- 3 tablespoons sesame oil

Instructions:

Over low heat, melt beeswax with water. Add cocoa butter. Stir until blended. Add the oils one at a time until well mixed. Store in an opaque glass jar and allow to cool. Smooth a small amount onto your skin.

Apricot-rose moisturi7

Ingredients:

- 2 tablespoons apricot kernel oil
- 1 tablespoon rosehip seed essential oil
- 1 tablespoon beeswax
- 1 teaspoon fennel oil
- 4 tablespoons rose water

Instructions:

Over low heat, melt oils with the beeswax. Allow to cool before slowly adding the rose water. Will store nicely in a dark, glass container with a tight lid for several days.

Creamy lime moisturizer

Ingredients:

- 1/4 cup milk
- Juice of one lime
- 2 tablespoons extra virgin olive oil

Instructions:

Boil milk and add other ingredients. Mix well and allow to cool before applying to your face. Refrigerate any extras for up to a week.

Grape-citrus moisturizer

Ingredients:

- 5 red or green grapes
- 2 teaspoons lemon, lime or orange juice
- 1 tablespoon oil of your choice

Instructions:

Whip until smooth in a food processor and apply a thin layer to skin. Refrigerator any extras for up to a week.

Honey-coconut moisturizer

Ingredients:

- 1 tablespoon coconut oil
- 1 teaspoon lemon juice
- 1 teaspoon honey

Instructions:

Mix all ingredients well and apply to dry skin. You can leave this moisturizer on for several hours or rinse off with warm water. You can refrigerate leftovers for a week.

Cucumber-lime moisturizer

Ingredients:

- 1 small cucumber, peeled, seeded
- Juice of one lime
- 2 tablespoons almond oil

Instructions:

Mix all ingredients in a food processor. Can be left on the skin for a few hours before rinsing off with warm water. Save any extra in the refrigerator for up to three days.

Creamy citrus moisturizer

Ingredients:

- 1 tablespoon each lemon juice and orange juice
- 1/2 cup yogurt

Instructions:

Mix well and leave on for up to a few hours before rinsing with warm water.

Milk & egg moisturizer

Ingredients:

- 1 large egg yolk
- 1/4 cup whole milk
- 1 tablespoon grapeseed oil

Instructions:

Mix all ingredients together until it is the consistency of a cream. Apply daily to the skin. Will stay fresh for a few days if kept in the refrigerator.

Honey-oat moisturizer

Ingredients:

- 1 tablespoon honey
- 1/8 cup cooked oatmeal
- 1/2 tablespoon aloe vera gel squeezed from a fresh leaf

Instructions:

Mix all ingredients well and apply to skin for 30 minutes before rinsing with warm water.

Nighttime rose moisturizer

Ingredients:

- 2 tablespoon rose petals
- 1/4 cup dried nonfat milk
- 4 tablespoons extra virgin olive oil

Instructions:

Blend all ingredients in a food processor and strain. Apply a small amount before going to bed.

Chapter 6: Facial Mask Recipes

The beauty of making facial masks at home are that not only do they cost mere pennies, but they can also be made from everyday ingredients that have amazingly strong benefits for your skin.

The facial masks that you will make contain thickly textured ingredients, like mashed avocados or bananas, as well as other fruits or vegetables. These ingredients give the mask some heft, but they also provide a ton of skin-boosting nutrients.

Avocados have lots of vitamin E and are considered a great ingredient to include if you have dry skin. Carrots provide a good dose of beta-carotene, which has been shown to improve skin's coloring. Both ingredients also work to help boost collagen production.

Facial masks are used occasionally (once or twice a week) to give the skin a deep cleaning and remove dirt, makeup, and toxins from the skin. This is why fruit like strawberries are often used, thanks to their astringent qualities. A vegetable like pumpkin will work as a gentle scrub that is not abrasive. However, it may cause some slight tingling. Masks with a clay base will also help to draw out impurities in the skin.

Some facial masks provide significant moisturizing for the skin with the use of light oils, such as almond, which absorb easily into the skin, softening and nourishing it. These oils are often paired with honey, with is a natural hydrator. It is also ideal for oily skin types because it helps to retain moisture without having to worry about the mystery ingredients in store-bought products.

Masks that include citrus fruits or apples may help to tone and lighten the skin if dark spots have occurred during the aging process.

To get the correct consistency in these masks, you may need to cook some of the ingredients and mash them. Be sure the ingredient has cooled completely before you apply it to your face. You can also store these masks for a few days in your refrigerator if you have leftovers. Do not use them after three or four days, as they will begin to spoil.

It is best to use a facial mask on clean skin so that the ingredients can be well absorbed. After you use and remove the mask, follow with a toner and moisturizer. You can use a mask once or twice a week, but don't use them on the same days that you use your exfoliating scrub as you may strip too many of the natural oils from your skin.

Occasional but regular use of both masks and scrubs will help to keep your pores free of dirt and dead skin cells and will reveal youthful skin that has a healthy glow to it. You may even start to notice that you have fewer fine lines and wrinkles.

Don't forget that these masks can also be applied to dry, or chapped, hands and feet, which may also need some extra attention, especially during the winter months.

Egg white face mask

Ingredients:

- 2 egg whites
- 2 tablespoons plain yogurt

Instructions:

Mix egg whites and yogurt well and apply to face. Rinse with warm water after 10 minutes.

Milk mask for dry skin

Ingredients:

- 1/2 teaspoon dry milk
- 1/2 tablespoon honey
- 1/2 teaspoon aloe vera gel
- 1 drop essential oil of your choice

Instructions:

Mix all ingredients well and apply to face for 15 minutes before rinsing off with warm water.

Applesauce mask

Ingredients:

- 1 tablespoon wheat germ
- 1 tablespoon applesauce (unflavored)

Instructions:

Blend ingredients together until they make a paste. Apply to freshly washed skin and leave on for 15 minutes. Rinse with warm water.

Avocado-carrot mask

Ingredients:

- 3 tablespoons honey
- 1/2 cup heavy cream
- 1 mashed avocado
- 1 cooked and mashed carrot
- 1 egg, beaten

Instructions:

Combine all ingredients until well mixed. Spread the mixture on your face and neck and let set for 15 minutes before rinsing with cool water.

Pumpkin mask

Ingredients:

- 1 egg
- 1 cup canned pumpkin
- 1 fresh papaya, mashed

Instructions:

Beat the egg until it is frothy, then add papaya and mix well. Mix in the pumpkin next until well blended. Apply to cleansed skin, avoiding the eye area. Leave on for 10 minutes and then rinse with warm water.

Banana mask

Ingredients:

- 1 egg white
- 1 tablespoon plain yogurt
- 1/2 teaspoon of your preferred oil (jojoba or grapeseed)
- 1 tablespoon honey
- 1 tablespoon white clay
- 1 ripe mashed banana

Instructions:

Whisk the egg white and add yogurt, oil, honey and clay. Mix until creamy. Add mashed banana and mix well. Massage into skin and leave on for 15 minutes. Rinse with warm water.

Kelp mask

Ingredients:

- 3 tablespoons plain yogurt
- 1 teaspoon powdered kelp
- 1 teaspoon honey

Instructions:

Mix yogurt and kelp until well blended, then add honey and mix. Apply to a clean face and neck. Leave on for 15 minutes before rinsing with a warm washcloth.

Rose-honey mask

Ingredients:

- 1 tablespoon honey
- 1 tablespoon almond oil
- 3 drops rose essential oil
- 1 drop vitamin E oil

Instructions:

Mix all ingredients well and apply to clean face and neck. Leave on for 15 minutes before removing with a warm washcloth.

Yogurt-honey mask

Ingredients:

- 1 tablespoon honey
- 1 tablespoon plain yogurt

Instructions:

Mix honey and yogurt well. Apply right after cleansing. Leave on for 10 minutes and rinse with warm water.

Fruit and honey mask

Ingredients:

- 1 cup strawberries, mashed
- 1 teaspoon lemon juice
- 2 egg whites
- 3 teaspoons honey
- 2-3 drops of essential oil of your choice

Instructions:

Mix all ingredients together until smooth. Apply a generous amount over face and neck and let set for 10 minutes before rinsing with warm water.

Chapter 7: Facial Toner Recipes

The role of a toner is to create the right balance of natural oils and moisture in your skin. If you have particularly dry skin, you may be able to do without a toner, but those with oily or combination skin may find that a toner helps to control blemishes and pH balance.

Toners are typically lightweight liquids that are applied with a cotton ball. Over-the-counter toners often contain alcohol as an astringent. It can be very drying and irritating, however, to many types of skin, even the most oily skin. Many natural ingredients provide antiseptic and astringent qualities—certain fruit juices and herbs, for example. Keep in mind, that because natural ingredients can also do some deep cleansing, your homemade toner may be drying. It may be a better option to use your toner only once a day.

When seeped in hot water, the tea made from herbs can be used to create liquid toners that are great for cleaning and tightening the skin, while reducing under-eye puffiness, and even lessening irritation from inflamed skin. Rosemary, which helps renew cells, is a good astringent, as is Thyme.

Other ingredients, like aloe vera, have healing properties that can be beneficial to skin that is prone to acne. Vinegar is a natural ingredient that will clean pores while helping to restore the skin's delicate balance.

You may be surprised to see white wine in the list of ingredients, but it contains an ingredient called alpha-hydroxy, which can stimulate healthy cell growth. Witch hazel has been used for centuries to cure skin diseases, and is a common ingredient in natural toners. You can find it at many drug stores or health food stores.

If you have sensitive skin, dab a bit of the recipe you want to try onto the inside of your elbow, then wait for 24 hours to see if you have a reaction. If a reaction occurs, do not use it on your face. Try experimenting with other ingredients that may not cause your skin to react.

If you opt for making your own rose water by heating rose petals in water, be sure to choose roses that have not been sprayed with pesticides. That said, rose water can help skin to feel refreshed and will also help to achieve pH balance.

Most of these toner recipes can be saved in the refrigerator for a few days in a container with a tight lid. You can also mix them up and pour them into ice cube trays, and then thaw them as you need them. If you use an essential oil, it may separate after sitting for a while. Simply shake the mixture well before using.

You will want to use a toner soon after your cleanse your skin. Then, while your skin is still slightly damp, apply your moisturizer directly after the toner. Be sure to avoid the skin around your eyes when applying a toner.

Wine & herb toner

Ingredients:

- 1 cup white wine
- 1 teaspoon dried rosemary
- 1 teaspoon dried thyme
- 1 teaspoon fresh mint leaves, chopped

Instructions:

Simmer ingredients over low heat for 10 minutes. Remove from heat and let set for an hour. Strain liquid, discard herbs and store in a bottle with a tight lid.

Cucumber toner

Ingredients:

- 1 cucumber, peeled and chopped
- 2 teaspoons honey

Instructions:

Use a blender to puree a cumber, and then put cucumber puree through a sieve. Add the honey to the clear cucumber juice. Shake bottle well and apply to skin with a cotton pad. You can save this toner in the refrigerator for a week.

Honey-lemon toner

Ingredients:

- 1 egg white
- 1 teaspoon honey
- 1 teaspoon lemon juice

Instructions:

Whisk egg white until it gets frothy, then add the honey and lemon juice. Apply to skin with a cotton pad and leave on for 10 minutes before rinsing with warm water.

Tomato-honey toner

Ingredients:

- 3 tablespoons tomato juice (preferably fresh)
- 1 teaspoon honey

Instructions:

Blend together and apply to face and neck. Rinse with warm water.

Cucumber-carrot toner

Ingredients:

- 1 tablespoon fresh mint leaves, whole
- 4 tablespoons cucumber juice
- 2 tablespoons carrot juice
- juice of one lemon

Instructions:

Make a strong mint tea by pouring boiling water over the mint leaves. Let seep for a few minutes, then remove leaves and allow to cool. Mix cooled tea with other ingredients and apply with a cotton pad.

Herbal toner

Ingredients:

- 2 sprigs of fresh thyme or 1/2 tablespoon dried thyme
- 2 teaspoons crushed fennel seeds
- 1/2 cup boiling water
- 1 tablespoon freshly squeezed lemon juice

Instructions:

Pour boiling water over thyme and fennel seeds. Add lemon juice and let set for 15 minutes. Strain and store in the refrigerator for no more than a week.

Fruity toner

Ingredients:

- 1 papaya, peeled, seeded and chopped
- 4 tablespoons apple cider vinegar

Instructions:

Place papaya in food processor and liquefy. Add vinegar and mix well. Keeps well in the refrigerator for up to a week.

Refreshing mint toner

Ingredients:

- 1/2 cup witch hazel
- 1/8 cup white wine vinegar
- 1/8 teaspoon mint extract
- 3-4 mint leaves

Instructions:

Mix ingredients well and store in a glass bottle. Apply with a cotton ball.

Aloe toner

Ingredients:

- 1 tablespoons Aloe vera gel
- 1/2 teaspoon lime juice

Instructions:

Blend the gel and juice together until mixed well. Use a cotton pad to apply to the skin.

Rose toner

Ingredients:

- 2 tablespoons rose water
- 1/4 tablespoon alum
- 1.75 oz glycerine

Instructions:

Mix ingredients well and apply with a cotton pad. Store mixture in refrigerator for up to three days.

Chapter 8: Facial Scrub Recipes

The role that facial scrubs play is to remove stubborn dirt and grime that has taken hold in your skin's pores, making you more susceptible to breakouts, dryness, and even premature wrinkles. You can tell that you have clogged pores if you have small blackheads, typically across your nose, or tiny white bumps that can be found anywhere on your face.

Clogged pores, however, are not always so obvious. Sometimes they will just make your skin appear dull and lifeless. Regularly examining your skin will help you to better determine when you might need a scrub. Ironically, some facial products that promise to produce healthier skin may actually clog your pores, especially if they contain mineral oil. Some shampoos and conditioners that contain a lot of chemicals will cause clogged pores around your hairline, causing pimples.

An effective facial scrub will include an ingredient that is somewhat abrasive in order to work on a deeper level. Many of the facial scrubs you will find on the market these days actually use a lot of wholesome ingredients, like sea salt, sugar, and ground almonds, as their exfoliating forces. However, most of them also include tiny, perfectly round chemical beads that do the work.

For a fraction of the price you can make your own facial scrub that works without harsh chemicals, often smells fantastic, and leaves you with beautifully renewed skin.

Some of the typical exfoliating ingredients you will see are salt, which can help to remove dry skin patches, sugar, used to reduce blemishes, and other ground ingredients that not only clean out your pores, but also offer some antioxidant and anti-inflammatory properties. You will need to mix these with a liquid of some sort before applying the scrub to your skin—usually an oil or honey.

When you use your scrub, it should feel mildly abrasive, but it should not be uncomfortable. If it feels too harsh, you may want to switch to another scrubbing ingredient. Oatmeal is a very gentle and effective scrub ingredient. Baking soda is another gentle exfoliant that has been proven to help remove blackheads, but is not gritty like salt or sugar can be.

Most of these recipes are meant for just one application. If you have extra, give them to a neighbor or store in the refrigerator for a day or two—but not longer.

You will want to use a scrub only once or twice a week, after you clean your face, but before you moisturize. Since the recipes already include an abrasive ingredient, you do not need to apply a lot of pressure when you are massaging the scrub into your skin. Just make small circles with your fingertips. It is best to do this when your skin is warm, like while you are in the shower. Don't forget to scrub your neck, chest, and back, as pores in these areas are susceptible to getting clogged.

Coffee scrub

Ingredients:

- 3 tablespoons brewed coffee grounds
- 1 tablespoon sea salt

Instructions:

Mix the grounds and salt and use within 20 minutes of brewing the coffee. You can use this scrub on your face and over your entire body.

Orange scrub

Ingredients:

- 1/2 a fresh orange
- 4 tablespoons cornmeal

Instructions:

Squeeze the juice and pulp of the orange into a bowl and mix with cornmeal until it creates a paste. Scrub gently into the face for two minutes and rinse.

Almond scrub

Ingredients:

- 2 tablespoons almond flour
- 1 tablespoons jojoba oil (or other oil of your choice)
- 2 tablespoons honey
- 2 drops of peppermint essential oil

Instructions:

Stir almond flour and oil in a dark glass container. Mix in honey and essential oil. To use, scoop some of the scrub into your hand and add a few drops of water before gently massaging into your face, neck and chest. Rinse with warm water.

Oatmeal scrub

Ingredients:

- 2 teaspoons ground oatmeal
- 1 teaspoon baking soda

Instructions:

Mix ingredients and add a small amount of distilled water to make a paste. Massage into face and neck before rinsing with warm water.

Apple scrub

Ingredients:

- 1 tablespoon white sugar
- 2 tablespoons applesauce
- 1 tablespoon olive oil (or oil of your choice)

Instructions:

Mix all ingredients together and gently massage into face for one to two minutes. Rinse well.

Pumpkin-sugar scrub

Ingredients:

- 1/2 cup canned pumpkin
- 1/2 cup brown sugar
- 1/4 teaspoon ground cinnamon

Instructions:

Mix ingredients well and apply to face and body—wherever you want to slough away dry skin. Rinse with warm water.

Wholesome scrub

Ingredients:

- 2 teaspoons wheat bran
- 2 tablespoons oatmeal
- 2 tablespoons olive oil
- 1 teaspoon dried parsley

Instructions:

Blend all ingredients in a food processor until well mixed and the desired consistency.

Sea salt scrub

Ingredients:

- 1/2 cup grapeseed oil
- 1 cup finely ground sea salt
- 5 drops of desired essential oil, such as lavender or rosemary

Instructions:

Mix oil and salt until it reaches the desired consistency, then add a few drops of essential oil at a time. Massage for a minute into skin before rinsing.

Sugar scrub

Ingredients:

- 1/4 cup white sugar
- 1/4 cup light brown sugar
- 1 teaspoon vanilla extract
- 1 teaspoon jojoba oil
- 1 tablespoon honey

Instructions:

Mix sugars, then add next three ingredients one at a time. Gently massage into your face and rinse. Store extras in a dark glass jar with a tight lid.

Simple brown sugar scrub

Ingredients:

- 1/2 cup brown sugar
- 1/4 cup olive oil

Instructions:

Mix ingredients together and rub gently into the face in small circles. Rinse well with warm water.

Chapter 9: Eye Treatment Recipes

Eye creams are a big business, and that is because the skin around the eyes is more susceptible to the effects of aging, lifestyle choices, and environmental stress than any other region. This delicate skin reacts in many, many ways. The first effects to appear are typically dark circles and puffiness (although these can also occur because of genetics, lack of internal hydration, and lack of sleep). Fine lines and wrinkles are next, followed by droopy eyelids that can make the eyes look tired when you may not be.

While this skin shows the signs of distress, it can also react dramatically to certain skincare products—and not always in a good way. When using any sort of moisturizer, toner, mask, or scrub, it is essential to stay away from the eye area, since it can react negatively.

The skin around your eyes should have its own, special treatments to counteract dark circles, puffiness, and aging skin. When creating your homemade eye creams, look for gentle ingredients such as rose water, ripe fruits, herbs, and certain vegetables that can ease under-eye puffiness.

Be sure to test any formulas that you make on the skin inside your elbow to determine if you skin will have a negative reaction. You do not want to experiment on the skin around your eyes, as you may be very uncomfortable until the effects wear off.

When applying your recipes to the eye area skin, use a gentle, patting motion with your ring finger. This is because the ring finger is generally used less and often has a softer surface. Also, it will not exert as much pressure as your pointer or middle finger would. Do not pull or tug on the skin.

If you don't have time to whip up a recipe, you can place two chilled cucumber slices or two chilled seeped tea bags on your eyes. Both of these will help to relieve puffiness—at least temporarily. You can also soak a cotton ball with milk and apply it under your eyes to reduce dark circles.

Another way to quickly reduce under-eye bags is to chill a spoon and place the back of it on your under-eye skin. Be careful with this method because if the spoon is too cold your skin may get red. You can also chill a gel pack that is made specifically for tired eyes.

Rose eye tonic

Ingredients:

- 1 oz rose water
- 8 oz distilled water

Instructions:

Mix rose water and distilled water in a large bowl and scoop some into your palms. Rinse your eyes whenever needed.

Pineapple-spice eye cream

Ingredients:

- 1 teaspoon turmeric powder
- 2 teaspoons pineapple juice

Instructions:

Make a fine paste with the turmeric and juice and apply under eyes. Leave on for 15 minutes before rinsing will cool water.

Almond eye cream

Ingredients:

- 1 teaspoon almond powder
- 2 teaspoons whole milk

Instructions:

Combine both ingredients and apply under the eyes for 20 minutes to reduce dark circles. Rinse with cool water.

Peach pulp

Ingredients:

- 1 peach or papaya, mashed

Instructions:

Continue to mash the fruit's pulp until it is a thick, pasty texture. Apply it under your eyes and leave it for 20 minutes before you wash it off with cool water.

Lemon paste

Ingredients:

- 1 teaspoon tomato juice
- 2 teaspoons lemon juice
- 1 teaspoon turmeric powder

Instructions:

Mix all ingredients into a fine paste and allow it to dry. Rinse off with cool water.

Rosemary eye cream

Ingredients:

- 1 sprig of rosemary leaf
- 3 oz boiling water
- 1 teaspoon ground almonds
- 1 tablespoon egg white

Instructions:

Make a tea with the rosemary leaf and boiling water. Allow to cool and remove leaf. Mix 2 tablespoons of the rosemary tea with the almonds and egg white. Gently pat some of the mixture under your eyes and allow to soak for 15 minutes. Rinse with warm water.

Eye wrinkle oil

Ingredients:

- 1 oz jojoba oil
- 5 drops chamomile essential oil
- 5 drops rose essential oil

Instructions:

Combine all oils and store in a small glass bottle with a tight lid. Apply a drop on your fingertip and gently pat into skin around the eye, except the eyelid.

Cucumber gel

Ingredients:

- 1 tablespoon aloe vera gel
- 1 teaspoon cucumber juice
- 1/4 teaspoon cornstarch
- 1 tablespoon witch hazel

Instructions:

Mix gel, juice and cornstarch over low heat until it just begins to boil. Remove from heat and add witch hazel. Once cooled, it will have a gel-like texture. To use, pat some under your eyes. Store in a small jar and keep away from the sunlight.

Apple-potato eye cream

Ingredients:

- 1 small potato
- 2 tablespoons unsweetened applesauce

Instructions:

Coarsely grind the potato and mix in the applesauce. Gently apply under the eyes and top with a warm washcloth. Take a rest for 5-10 minutes before washing off with warm water.

Avocado eye cream

Ingredients:

- 1 slice of avocado
- drizzle of almond oil

Instructions:

Mix the ingredients to desired texture and apply under and around the eyes. Let set for 10 minutes before rinsing with warm water.

Made in the USA
Middletown, DE
19 November 2018